# The Brighter Side of Dentistry: Cosmetic Procedures for Students

**HENRY**

# Water for Life:

# The Brighter Side of Dentistry: Cosmetic Procedures for Students

# Copyright © 2023 by HENRY



**The first edition was published in 2023**

**ISBN**:
Published by:
Sunshine
1663 Liberty Drive
Hyderabad, IN 47403
www.Sunshinepublishers.com

**This book is self-published using on-demand printing and publishing, which allows it to be printed and distributed globally**

# TABLE OF CONTENT

## Chapter 1: Introduction to Cosmetic Dentistry for Students



The Importance of a Bright Smile

Understanding Cosmetic Dentistry

Benefits of Cosmetic Dentistry for Students

## Chapter 2: Common Cosmetic Procedures for Students



Teeth Whitening: Brightening Your Smile

Dental Veneers: Perfecting Your Teeth's Appearance

Dental Implants: Restoring Your Confidence

## Chapter 3: Preparing for Cosmetic Procedures as a Student



Finding the Right Cosmetic Dentist

Understanding the Procedure Process

Financial Considerations and Insurance Options

# Chapter 1: Introduction to Cosmetic Dentistry for Students

## The Importance of a Bright Smile

A smile is a powerful tool that can brighten someone's day, make a lasting impression, and boost your confidence. As students, it is crucial to understand the significance of maintaining a bright, healthy smile. In this subchapter, we will delve into the importance of a bright smile and how it relates to the field of dentistry.

First and foremost, a bright smile is aesthetically pleasing and can enhance your overall appearance. When you have a healthy set of pearly whites, it can help you feel more confident in social situations, whether it be presenting in front of your classmates or connecting with new friends. A bright smile can make you feel more approachable and leave a positive impression on those you interact with.

Moreover, a bright smile is an indicator of good oral health. Healthy teeth and gums are crucial for proper chewing and digestion. When you take care of your oral hygiene, you reduce the risk of developing cavities, gum disease, and other dental issues. Regular brushing, flossing, and dental check-ups are essential habits to maintain a bright and healthy smile.

Additionally, a bright smile can have a significant impact on your professional life. In the field of dentistry, a bright smile is not only a reflection of your oral health but also a symbol of your expertise. As students aspiring to work in the dental field, it is crucial to understand the importance of leading by example. By taking care of your own smile, you demonstrate to future patients the significance of oral hygiene and the positive outcomes it can bring.

Furthermore, a bright smile can boost your self-esteem and overall well-being. When you have a healthy smile, you are more likely to feel confident and comfortable in your own skin. This confidence can extend to all aspects of your life, including academics, relationships, and personal growth.

In conclusion, a bright smile is not only visually appealing but also an essential aspect of good oral health, professional success, and personal well-being. As students in the field of dentistry, it is important to understand the significance of maintaining a bright smile and leading by example. By prioritizing oral hygiene and taking care of your own smile, you can inspire others to do the same and make a positive impact in the world of dentistry. Remember, a bright smile is not just a cosmetic feature, but a reflection of your overall health and happiness.

## Understanding Cosmetic Dentistry

Cosmetic dentistry has become increasingly popular in recent years, as more and more people strive to achieve the perfect smile. But what exactly is cosmetic dentistry, and how does it differ from traditional dentistry? In this subchapter, we will delve into the world of cosmetic dentistry and explore the various procedures that can help enhance your smile.

Cosmetic dentistry is a branch of dentistry that focuses on improving the appearance of teeth, gums, and overall smile. Unlike traditional dentistry, which primarily focuses on the health and functionality of teeth, cosmetic dentistry aims to enhance the aesthetics. It involves various procedures that can correct imperfections such as discoloration, misalignment, gaps, chips, and more.

One of the most common cosmetic dentistry procedures is teeth whitening. This procedure helps to remove stains and discoloration, resulting in a brighter and more youthful smile. Teeth whitening can be done in-office or at home using special bleaching agents under the supervision of a dentist.

Another popular procedure is dental veneers. Veneers are thin, custom-made shells that are bonded to the front surface of teeth. They can be used to correct a range of imperfections, including chips, cracks, and gaps. Veneers can also improve the shape and alignment of teeth, giving you a flawless smile.

For those with crooked or misaligned teeth, orthodontic treatments such as braces or clear aligners can help. Braces use metal brackets and wires to gradually shift teeth into their desired position, while clear aligners are removable and virtually invisible, making them a more discreet option.

Cosmetic dentistry also offers solutions for missing teeth, such as dental implants and bridges. Dental implants are artificial tooth roots that are surgically placed into the jawbone, providing a strong foundation for replacement teeth. Bridges, on the other hand, are used to fill the gap left by missing teeth and are anchored to the adjacent teeth.

In conclusion, cosmetic dentistry is a specialized field that focuses on improving the appearance of teeth and enhancing smiles. From teeth whitening to dental veneers, braces, and dental implants, there is a wide range of procedures available to help you achieve the smile of your dreams. By understanding cosmetic dentistry, students can gain insight into the importance of aesthetics in dentistry and the various techniques used to enhance smiles.

# Benefits of Cosmetic Dentistry for Students

In today's image-conscious society, having a bright and confident smile is more important than ever. As students, our appearance plays a significant role in our confidence and self-esteem. This is where cosmetic dentistry comes into the picture, offering a range of procedures that can enhance our smiles and improve our overall dental health. In this subchapter, we will explore the numerous benefits of cosmetic dentistry for students.

First and foremost, cosmetic dentistry can greatly improve the aesthetics of our smiles. Whether it's teeth whitening, dental bonding, or veneers, these procedures can help us achieve a brighter and more attractive smile. As students, having a captivating smile can boost our self-confidence, making us feel more comfortable when interacting with peers, teachers, and potential employers.

Moreover, cosmetic dentistry can correct various dental issues that may affect our oral health. Misaligned teeth, gaps, or overcrowding can lead to difficulty in cleaning and maintaining good oral hygiene. By opting for orthodontic treatments like braces or clear aligners, students can achieve a straighter smile, reducing the risk of tooth decay, gum disease, and other dental problems.

Cosmetic dentistry can also provide long-term benefits for students. Dental implants, for instance, can replace missing teeth, restoring both functionality and aesthetics. This can prevent further oral health complications that may arise due to gaps in the dental structure. Additionally, certain cosmetic procedures, such as dental contouring or reshaping, can improve the alignment of the bite, reducing the risk of jaw pain and temporomandibular joint disorders.

Furthermore, investing in cosmetic dentistry as a student can have a positive impact on future endeavors. A beautiful smile can make a lasting impression during job interviews or social interactions, increasing our chances of success in both personal and professional aspects of life. Additionally, taking care of our dental health at a young age through cosmetic dentistry can prevent more extensive and costly treatments in the future.

In conclusion, cosmetic dentistry offers numerous benefits for students in terms of aesthetics, oral health, and overall confidence. By investing in our smiles, we can enhance our self-esteem, improve our dental health, and set a foundation for a successful future. So, let us embrace the brighter side of dentistry and unlock the potential of our smiles!

# Chapter 2: Common Cosmetic Procedures for Students

## Teeth Whitening: Brightening Your Smile

In this subchapter, we will explore the fascinating world of teeth whitening and how it can help you achieve a brighter and more confident smile. As students in the field of dentistry, it is essential to understand the various cosmetic procedures available to enhance oral aesthetics, and teeth whitening is a popular and effective option.

Why is teeth whitening important? A bright smile not only boosts your self-esteem but also leaves a lasting impression on others. Our teeth can become discolored over time due to various factors such as consuming highly pigmented foods and beverages, smoking, poor oral hygiene, or natural aging. Teeth whitening procedures can help reverse these effects, giving you a radiant smile that reflects good oral health.

There are several teeth whitening methods available today, ranging from over-the-counter products to professional treatments performed by dentists. Over-the-counter options, such as whitening toothpaste or strips, can be a convenient starting point for those on a budget. However, it is crucial to note that these products may not provide the same level of effectiveness as professional treatments.

Professional teeth whitening treatments, carried out by dentists, offer superior results and are tailored to individual needs. They involve the application of bleaching agents directly on the teeth, which effectively removes stains and discoloration. Dentists use various techniques like chairside bleaching, where a high-concentration bleaching gel is applied under controlled conditions, or take-home kits with custom-made trays for gradual whitening over a few weeks.

It is important to consult a dentist before undergoing any teeth whitening procedure. They will evaluate your oral health, identify potential risks, and recommend the most suitable treatment option for you. Additionally, dentists can provide valuable advice on maintaining your newly whitened smile, including proper oral hygiene practices and dietary modifications.

While teeth whitening can significantly enhance your smile, it is essential to remember that it is not a one-time process. The results of teeth whitening treatments are not permanent, and the longevity depends on various factors such as lifestyle choices and oral hygiene habits. Regular touch-ups and maintenance are necessary to keep your smile looking its best.

In conclusion, teeth whitening is a popular cosmetic procedure that can brighten your smile and boost your confidence. As students in the field of dentistry, it is crucial to understand the available teeth whitening methods and their benefits. By educating yourself about teeth whitening, you will be well-equipped to guide patients in achieving the smile they desire while maintaining good oral health. Remember, a brighter smile is just a whitening treatment away!

# Dental Veneers: Perfecting Your Teeth's Appearance

In the world of dentistry, there are countless procedures available to help enhance the appearance of our teeth. One such procedure that has gained immense popularity is dental veneers. Designed to perfect the appearance of your teeth, veneers offer a simple and effective solution for various dental imperfections. Whether you're dealing with chipped, stained, or misaligned teeth, veneers can help you achieve a brighter and more confident smile.

So, what exactly are dental veneers? Veneers are thin, custom-made shells made from tooth-colored materials such as porcelain or composite resin. These shells are bonded to the front surface of your teeth, covering any flaws and improving their overall appearance. The process typically involves two visits to your dentist, where they will assess your teeth, take impressions, and create your custom veneers.

One of the primary benefits of dental veneers is their ability to transform your smile in a relatively short amount of time. Unlike other procedures that may require several visits to the dentist, veneers can often be placed within a few weeks. This makes them an ideal option for students who are seeking a quick and effective solution to enhance their smile.

Furthermore, dental veneers are incredibly versatile. They can address a wide range of dental concerns, including gaps between teeth, misshapen or uneven teeth, and even stubborn discoloration that cannot be resolved through traditional teeth whitening methods. With veneers, you can achieve a natural-looking smile that is tailored to your specific needs and desires.

Additionally, veneers are known for their durability and longevity. With proper care and maintenance, they can last for many years, providing you with a beautiful smile for a long time. However, it is important to note that veneers are not indestructible and may require replacement over time.

In conclusion, dental veneers offer an excellent solution for students looking to perfect the appearance of their teeth. With their ability to address a wide range of dental imperfections and their quick and efficient process, veneers provide an effective way to enhance your smile. Consider consulting with your dentist to determine if dental veneers are the right option for you and take the first step towards achieving a brighter and more confident smile.

# Dental Implants: Restoring Your Confidence

In the world of dentistry, advancements in technology have made it possible to restore your smile and confidence like never before. One of the most groundbreaking procedures in modern dentistry is dental implants. For students studying dentistry, understanding the significance of dental implants is crucial as they will play a vital role in enhancing the lives of many patients.

So, what exactly are dental implants? Dental implants are artificial tooth roots that are surgically placed into the jawbone to provide a strong foundation for replacement teeth. Unlike dentures or bridges, dental implants are a permanent solution that look and feel like natural teeth. They offer a multitude of benefits, both aesthetically and functionally, making them a preferred choice for patients seeking a long-term solution for missing teeth.

From a cosmetic perspective, dental implants can greatly enhance a patient's self-confidence. Missing teeth can cause embarrassment and self-consciousness, impacting social interactions and overall well-being. With dental implants, individuals can regain their natural smile, allowing them to laugh, speak, and eat without feeling self-conscious. This restoration of confidence can have a profound impact on a person's life, positively influencing their relationships, career prospects, and overall happiness.

From a functional standpoint, dental implants offer significant advantages over other tooth replacement options. Traditional dentures can be uncomfortable, often slipping or clicking during speech and eating. Dental implants, on the other hand, are securely anchored in the jawbone, providing stability and durability that mimics natural teeth. This allows patients to eat their favorite foods without restrictions, enjoying a varied and healthy diet.

As students of dentistry, it is important to recognize the impact dental implants can have on a patient's quality of life. By understanding the procedure, its benefits, and its limitations, you will be better equipped to educate and guide your future patients towards making informed decisions about their dental health.

Furthermore, staying up-to-date with the latest advancements in dental implant technology will ensure that you provide the best possible care to your patients. As research continues to push the boundaries of what is possible, students of dentistry have the opportunity to contribute to the evolution of dental implant procedures and improve the lives of countless individuals.

In conclusion, dental implants have revolutionized the field of dentistry, offering a permanent and natural-looking solution for missing teeth. For students studying dentistry, understanding the significance of dental implants and their potential to restore confidence and improve quality of life is essential. By staying informed and embracing advancements in this field, you have the power to make a positive impact on the lives of your future patients.

# Chapter 3: Preparing for Cosmetic Procedures as a Student

## Finding the Right Cosmetic Dentist

When it comes to cosmetic dentistry, finding the right dentist is crucial to achieving the smile you desire. With so many options available, it can be overwhelming to choose the perfect dentist who understands your needs as a student. This subchapter will guide you through the essential factors to consider when searching for the right cosmetic dentist.

Firstly, it is important to look for a dentist who specializes in cosmetic dentistry. Not all dentists have the same level of expertise in this field, so finding someone who has extensive experience and knowledge in cosmetic procedures is key. Look for dentists who have undergone additional training or have certifications in cosmetic dentistry.

Secondly, consider the dentist's portfolio and before-and-after photos. This will give you a visual representation of their work and help you gauge their skill level. Pay attention to cases similar to your own, such as teeth whitening, veneers, or orthodontic treatments. By reviewing their previous work, you can get a sense of the dentist's aesthetic style and decide if it aligns with your own preferences.

Another crucial factor to consider is the dentist's reputation and patient reviews. Look for testimonials or online reviews from previous patients to get an idea of their overall satisfaction with the dentist's services. Positive reviews can provide reassurance and confidence in your choice, while negative reviews should be taken into consideration as well.

Accessibility and convenience should also be taken into account, especially as a busy student. Look for a dental office that is conveniently located near your campus or residence, with flexible appointment hours that can accommodate your schedule. Additionally, inquire about their payment options and whether they accept dental insurance, as this can greatly impact your overall experience.

Lastly, do not underestimate the importance of personal connection and comfort. A cosmetic dentist should be someone you can openly communicate with about your concerns and desires. Schedule a consultation with potential dentists to assess their communication skills and whether they listen to your needs attentively.

By considering these factors, you will be well on your way to finding the right cosmetic dentist who can help you achieve the smile of your dreams. Remember, investing in your dental appearance can have a significant impact on your confidence and overall well-being as a student.

## Understanding the Procedure Process

When it comes to dentistry, understanding the procedure process is essential for students who aspire to excel in this field. Whether you dream of becoming a dentist or dental hygienist, having a comprehensive understanding of the steps involved in various dental procedures is crucial. In this subchapter, we will delve into the procedure process, providing you with valuable insights into the world of dentistry.

First and foremost, it is essential to recognize that each dental procedure follows a systematic process. This process typically begins with a thorough examination and diagnosis of the patient's oral health. This step helps dental professionals identify any underlying issues and determine the most suitable treatment plan.

Once the diagnosis is complete, the next phase involves explaining the treatment plan to the patient. As students, you will learn how to effectively communicate with patients, ensuring they understand the procedure, its benefits, and any potential risks or complications.

The actual procedure begins with the preparation of the patient, which may involve administering anesthesia or sedation, depending on the complexity of the treatment. This step is vital in ensuring the patient's comfort during the procedure, as well as minimizing any pain or anxiety they may experience.

During the procedure itself, students will learn the intricacies of various dental treatments, such as tooth extractions, fillings, root canals, and cosmetic procedures like teeth whitening or veneers. Understanding the specific steps involved in each procedure, including the use of specialized tools and techniques, is crucial for achieving successful outcomes.

Post-procedure care is equally important, as it contributes to the overall success and satisfaction of the patient. Students will learn about proper aftercare instructions, including medications, oral hygiene practices, and potential complications to watch out for. It is crucial to educate patients on how to maintain their oral health post-procedure, ensuring long-lasting results.

Throughout this subchapter, we will explore various dental procedures, breaking down the process and providing valuable tips and insights to help you succeed in your dental career. By understanding the procedure process, students can develop the necessary skills and knowledge to provide exceptional dental care to their future patients.

Remember, dentistry is not merely about technical skills; it also requires empathy, communication, and a genuine passion for helping others. So, dive into this subchapter, absorb the knowledge, and prepare yourself for a rewarding journey into the brighter side of dentistry.

# Financial Considerations and Insurance Options

As students pursuing a career in dentistry, it is essential to understand the financial considerations and insurance options associated with the field. While the primary focus may be on learning and honing your dental skills, it is equally important to be well-informed about the financial aspects of your future profession. This subchapter aims to provide you with valuable insights into managing your finances and exploring insurance options as a dental student.

First and foremost, it is crucial to have a realistic understanding of the financial commitments that come with being a dentist. Dental school can be expensive, with tuition fees, textbooks, and other educational expenses. Keeping a budget and seeking financial aid opportunities, such as scholarships and grants, can help alleviate some of the financial burdens.

Additionally, it is important to consider the long-term financial implications of establishing your own dental practice. Starting a practice requires significant upfront investment, including equipment, office space, and staff. Understanding the financial aspects of practice ownership, including managing overhead costs, setting fees, and planning for retirement, is essential.

Insurance is another critical aspect of financial planning for dental students. As a future dentist, you will need to consider various insurance options to protect yourself, your practice, and your patients. Professional liability insurance, also known as malpractice insurance, is a must-have for any practicing dentist. This insurance coverage protects you in case of any claims or lawsuits resulting from patient dissatisfaction or alleged negligence.

Additionally, you should carefully evaluate other insurance options, such as disability insurance and business insurance, to safeguard your financial stability and protect your practice from unforeseen circumstances. Disability insurance provides income replacement in the event that you are unable to work due to illness or injury, ensuring financial security during challenging times.

Lastly, it is essential to understand the role of dental insurance in your future practice. Familiarize yourself with different types of dental insurance plans, reimbursement models, and coding systems to effectively navigate the insurance landscape and optimize patient care. Understanding insurance options will allow you to provide quality dental services while maximizing reimbursement for your services.

In conclusion, financial considerations and insurance options play a vital role in the dental profession. As dental students, it is crucial to be well-informed about the financial commitments and insurance policies associated with dentistry. By managing your finances responsibly, exploring insurance options, and staying updated with the ever-evolving insurance landscape, you can ensure a bright and successful future in dentistry.

# Chapter 4: Taking Care of Your Teeth After Cosmetic Procedures

## Maintaining Oral Hygiene for Long-lasting Results

As students pursuing a career in dentistry, it is crucial to understand the importance of maintaining oral hygiene for long-lasting results. Oral health not only contributes to our overall well-being but also plays a significant role in our confidence and self-esteem. By establishing good oral hygiene habits early on, we can ensure a lifetime of healthy smiles for ourselves and our future patients.

The foundation of maintaining oral hygiene starts with regular and proper brushing. It is recommended to brush our teeth at least twice a day using fluoride toothpaste. Choosing a soft-bristled toothbrush and brushing in gentle, circular motions helps remove plaque and food particles effectively. Remember to replace your toothbrush every three to four months or when the bristles become frayed.

In addition to brushing, flossing is equally important. Dental floss reaches the areas between our teeth and along the gumline where toothbrushes cannot reach. By flossing daily, we can prevent the buildup of plaque and reduce the risk of gum disease and tooth decay. Make it a habit to floss before bedtime to remove any lingering food particles from the day.

Maintaining a healthy diet also significantly impacts our oral health. Limiting sugary and acidic foods and beverages can prevent tooth decay and enamel erosion. Opt for a balanced diet rich in fruits, vegetables, and calcium-rich foods like dairy products to promote strong teeth and gums.

Regular dental check-ups and cleanings are crucial for long-lasting oral health. As students, we should schedule routine visits with our dentists every six months. These appointments allow for early detection and prevention of dental issues. Professional cleanings help remove tartar buildup and provide a fresh start for maintaining oral hygiene.

Lastly, it is essential to be mindful of habits that can negatively impact our oral health. Avoid smoking or chewing tobacco, as these habits are known to cause oral cancer, gum disease, and tooth loss. Additionally, limit alcohol consumption, as it can contribute to dry mouth and tooth decay.

By following these oral hygiene practices consistently, we can ensure long-lasting results for ourselves and our future patients. As students in the field of dentistry, it is our responsibility to lead by example and educate others on the importance of maintaining oral hygiene. Together, we can promote healthy smiles and improve the overall oral health of our communities.

## Diet and Lifestyle Changes for Optimal Oral Health

Maintaining good oral health is not only crucial for a beautiful smile but also for overall well-being. As students pursuing a career in dentistry, it is essential to understand the significance of diet and lifestyle choices in promoting optimal oral health. By adopting healthy habits, you can not only prevent dental problems but also educate your future patients about the importance of oral hygiene. Let's explore some key diet and lifestyle changes that can contribute to a brighter and healthier smile.

1. Limit Sugary and Acidic Foods: Consuming excessive sugary and acidic foods can lead to tooth decay and enamel erosion. As future dental professionals, it's important to educate yourself and others about the harmful effects of these foods. Encourage your patients and peers to limit their intake of sugary snacks, carbonated drinks, and citrus fruits. Instead, promote alternatives like fresh fruits, vegetables, and dairy products that are rich in vitamins and minerals beneficial for oral health.

2. Practice Regular Brushing and Flossing: Good oral hygiene practices are the foundation of a healthy smile. Remind yourself and your patients to brush at least twice a day with fluoride toothpaste and floss daily to remove plaque and prevent gum disease. Emphasize the importance of using proper brushing and flossing techniques to ensure effective cleaning.

3. Avoid Tobacco and Alcohol: Tobacco and alcohol consumption are detrimental to oral health. As future dental professionals, encourage your peers and patients to

quit smoking and avoid excessive alcohol consumption. Educate them about the risks of oral cancer, gum disease, and tooth loss associated with these habits.

4. Stay Hydrated: Drinking an adequate amount of water throughout the day helps maintain saliva production, which is essential for neutralizing acids and washing away food particles. Encourage your patients to choose water over sugary beverages for better oral health.

5. Regular Dental Check-ups: Stress the importance of regular dental check-ups and cleanings to your patients. These visits allow early detection and prevention of dental issues. As students of dentistry, it's crucial to set an example by scheduling your own regular dental appointments.

By incorporating these diet and lifestyle changes into your own life and educating others about them, you are promoting optimal oral health within the dentistry field. Remember, prevention is always better than cure, and as future dental professionals, you have the power to inspire and guide others towards a brighter and healthier smile.

# Regular Dental Check-ups and Maintenance

Maintaining good oral health is essential for everyone, and students are no exception. As students, you may be busy with your studies and extracurricular activities, but neglecting your dental health can have serious consequences. This subchapter aims to educate and emphasize the importance of regular dental check-ups and maintenance in your daily routine.

Regular dental check-ups are crucial in preventing dental problems and maintaining a healthy smile. By visiting your dentist at least twice a year, you can identify any potential issues before they become major concerns. During these check-ups, your dentist will thoroughly examine your teeth, gums, and mouth, looking for signs of decay, gum disease, or any other dental conditions. Early detection allows for prompt treatment, preventing further damage and potential discomfort.

In addition to check-ups, maintaining a proper oral hygiene routine is vital. Brushing your teeth at least twice a day with fluoride toothpaste and using dental floss to clean between your teeth can help remove plaque and prevent cavities. It is also essential to limit sugary snacks and beverages, as they can contribute to tooth decay. By adopting these habits, you can ensure the long-term health of your teeth and gums.

Moreover, regular dental check-ups provide an opportunity for professional cleaning. Even with diligent brushing and flossing, plaque and tartar can still accumulate in hard-to-reach areas. Dental hygienists are skilled at removing these deposits, leaving your teeth clean and polished. This thorough cleaning can help prevent gum disease and maintain a bright smile.

Beyond the immediate benefits, regular dental check-ups and maintenance contribute to your overall well-being. Poor oral health has been linked to various systemic diseases such as heart disease and diabetes. By taking care of your teeth and gums, you are investing in your long-term health and reducing the risk of these serious conditions.

In conclusion, as students pursuing careers in dentistry, it is vital to prioritize your own dental health. Regular dental check-ups and maintenance are crucial in preventing oral health problems, identifying issues at an early stage, and maintaining a beautiful smile. By establishing good oral hygiene habits and visiting your dentist regularly, you can ensure a healthier future for yourself and your patients. Don't neglect your dental health – it's the key to the brighter side of dentistry.

# Chapter 5: Frequently Asked Questions about Cosmetic Dentistry for Students

**Will cosmetic procedures affect my daily routine as a student?**

As a student, you may be concerned about how cosmetic procedures will impact your daily routine. It's natural to have questions and uncertainties, but rest assured, cosmetic procedures in dentistry are designed to enhance your smile without disrupting your student life. In fact, they can have a positive impact on your overall well-being and self-confidence.

One of the most significant advantages of cosmetic dental procedures is their minimal impact on your daily routine. Unlike more invasive treatments, such as orthodontics or oral surgery, many cosmetic procedures are quick and require little to no downtime. For example, teeth whitening can be done in a single visit, and you can resume your daily activities immediately afterward.

Additionally, cosmetic procedures like dental bonding or veneers can be completed in a few appointments, allowing you to plan accordingly and integrate them into your schedule. Your dentist will work with you to find the most convenient time slots, ensuring minimal disruption to your academic commitments.

Moreover, cosmetic dental procedures are tailored to fit your individual needs and desires. Your dentist will discuss your goals and expectations, considering your lifestyle and preferences. Whether you want a brighter smile, straighter teeth, or a complete smile makeover, the treatment plan will be designed to suit your unique situation. This means that your daily routine will not be significantly affected, as the procedures will be customized to seamlessly fit into your life as a student.

Furthermore, cosmetic procedures can have a positive impact on your confidence and self-esteem. As a student, feeling self-assured in your appearance can greatly enhance your social interactions and academic performance. A beautiful smile can boost your self-image, leading to increased motivation and a more positive attitude towards your studies.

In conclusion, cosmetic dental procedures can be easily integrated into your daily routine as a student. With their minimal impact on your schedule and the ability to customize the treatments to your specific needs, you can enjoy the benefits of an improved smile without sacrificing your academic commitments. Embracing cosmetic dentistry can not only enhance your appearance but also boost your self-confidence, ultimately contributing to your overall success as a student.

## Can I afford cosmetic dentistry as a student?

One of the common concerns among students considering cosmetic dentistry is the affordability factor. As a student, budget constraints are a reality, and it's important to understand how cosmetic dental procedures fit into your financial situation. Fortunately, there are options and strategies that can make cosmetic dentistry more accessible to students who aspire to enhance their smiles.

First and foremost, it's essential to recognize that cosmetic dentistry is not just about aesthetics but also about the overall dental health and well-being. Many cosmetic procedures can address functional issues, such as misaligned teeth, bite problems, and overcrowding, which can lead to long-term oral health problems if left untreated. Therefore, investing in cosmetic dentistry can also be seen as a long-term investment in your oral health.

When it comes to the financial aspect, there are a few avenues to explore. Start by consulting your dental insurance provider to understand what procedures may be covered under your policy. While cosmetic treatments may not always be covered, some insurance plans offer partial coverage for procedures like braces or Invisalign, which can help align your teeth and improve your smile.

Additionally, many dental schools or teaching institutions offer reduced-cost or discounted treatments to patients. These institutions often provide supervised treatments by dental students or residents, allowing you to receive quality care at a fraction of the cost. While the treatment process may take longer due to the educational nature of the setting, the savings can be significant.

Another option to consider is dental financing plans. Many dental offices offer flexible payment options, allowing you to spread the cost of your treatment over several months or even years. This can make cosmetic dentistry more manageable for students on a tight budget, as you can make affordable monthly payments rather than paying a lump sum upfront.

Lastly, it's important to have an open and honest conversation with your dentist about your financial situation. They may be able to suggest alternative treatment options that are more budget-friendly or recommend procedures that provide the most significant impact for your specific needs.

In conclusion, while affordability may be a concern for students considering cosmetic dentistry, there are ways to make it more accessible. By exploring insurance coverage, seeking treatments at teaching institutions, considering financing options, and communicating with your dentist, you can find a solution that aligns with both your dental health goals and your budget. Remember, investing in your smile is an investment in your overall well-being and confidence, which can have a positive impact on your academic and personal life.

**Are there any risks or side effects associated with cosmetic procedures for students?**

As students, we all strive to look our best and feel confident in our appearance. With the increasing popularity of cosmetic procedures, it's natural for us to wonder about the potential risks and side effects associated with these treatments, especially when it comes to dentistry. In this subchapter, we will explore the possible risks and side effects of cosmetic procedures for students, providing you with the information you need to make an informed decision.

When it comes to dental cosmetic procedures, it's essential to understand that any treatment, no matter how minor, carries some inherent risks. One of the most common risks associated with dental procedures is infection. Although rare, infection can occur if proper sterilization techniques are not followed or if the patient has a compromised immune system. It is crucial to choose a reputable dentist who adheres to strict sterilization protocols to minimize this risk.

Another potential side effect of cosmetic procedures is tooth sensitivity. Many cosmetic procedures, such as teeth whitening or dental bonding, can cause temporary sensitivity to hot or cold temperatures. This sensitivity usually subsides within a few days, but it's important to discuss this possibility with your dentist beforehand.

In some cases, cosmetic procedures may also lead to gum irritation or recession. This is more common with procedures like dental veneers or crowns, where the tooth structure needs to be altered. However, with proper treatment planning and execution by an experienced dentist, the risk of gum-related complications can be minimized.

It's also crucial to note that some cosmetic procedures, such as orthodontic treatments or dental implants, require a more significant investment of time and money. While these treatments can enhance your smile in the long run, it's important to consider the commitment and potential discomfort associated with them before making a decision.

In conclusion, cosmetic procedures for students do come with some risks and side effects. However, these risks can be minimized by choosing a reputable dentist, discussing your concerns beforehand, and following post-treatment instructions. By being well-informed and taking necessary precautions, you can enjoy the benefits of a beautiful smile without compromising your oral health. Remember to always consult with a dental professional to determine the best course of action for your specific needs and desires.

# Chapter 6: Success Stories from Students who Underwent Cosmetic Dentistry

**Sharing Inspiring Stories of Transformation and Confidence Boost**

In the world of dentistry, the power to transform lives is not only limited to fixing smiles and providing oral health care. It goes beyond the physical aspect, reaching deep into the realm of self-confidence and personal growth. This subchapter aims to shed light on the inspiring stories of transformation and confidence boost that dentistry has brought to countless individuals, particularly students like you who are venturing into this field.

Imagine a young dental student, filled with passion and enthusiasm, but struggling with their own self-esteem. Meet Lisa, a bright and talented student who dreamed of becoming a dentist since childhood. However, she was plagued by insecurities due to her dental imperfections. Lisa had misaligned teeth and an uneven smile, which made her hesitant to speak up during class or engage in social interactions. Deep down, she knew that her dream of becoming a successful dentist would remain unfulfilled unless she addressed her own dental concerns.

With the support of her professors and mentors, Lisa embarked on a transformative journey. She underwent cosmetic dental procedures that corrected her misaligned teeth and enhanced her smile. As her dental issues were resolved, Lisa's confidence soared to new heights. She became a vocal participant in class discussions, took on leadership roles within her dental school, and even started mentoring other students who were going through similar struggles. Lisa's transformation not only improved her own self-esteem but also inspired others around her.

Similarly, we have Alex, a dental student who faced challenges with public speaking and patient interaction. Despite having a wealth of knowledge, Alex lacked the confidence to effectively communicate with patients, leading to missed opportunities for building trust and providing quality care. Determined to overcome this hurdle, Alex sought guidance from experienced dentists and communication experts. Through training and practice, Alex learned to speak with clarity, empathy, and confidence. This newfound ability not only transformed Alex's patient interactions but also elevated the quality of care being provided.

These stories of transformation and confidence boost highlight the power of dentistry to positively impact not only patients but also dental professionals themselves. As students, you have the unique opportunity to witness and be a part of these incredible journeys. By sharing these inspiring stories, we hope to ignite a fire within you, pushing you to believe in the transformative power of dentistry and the immense impact it can have on the lives of your future patients.

Remember, dentistry is not just about the technical skills; it is about the human connection and the ability to instill confidence and transform lives. Embrace the power of dentistry, and let these stories inspire you to become the best version of yourself, both personally and professionally.

## Overcoming Dental Challenges and Achieving Academic Success

Introduction:

As students pursuing a career in dentistry, we understand the unique challenges that come with balancing academic responsibilities and dental studies. However, it is important to remember that with determination and a positive mindset, you can overcome these challenges and achieve academic success. In this subchapter, we will discuss some common dental challenges faced by students and provide strategies for overcoming them.

Time Management:

One of the biggest challenges for dental students is managing their time effectively. With a demanding academic schedule, practical training, and extracurricular activities, it can be overwhelming to prioritize tasks. To excel academically, it is crucial to create a well-structured daily schedule. Set specific goals for each day and allocate time for studying, attending classes, and completing assignments. Prioritize tasks based on urgency and importance, and make sure to allocate time for self-care and relaxation.

Maintaining a Healthy Lifestyle:

Another challenge faced by dental students is maintaining a healthy lifestyle. The long hours of studying and practical training can often lead to neglecting personal health. However, it is important to prioritize self-care to excel academically. Make sure to get enough sleep, exercise regularly, and eat a balanced diet. Taking care of your physical and mental well-being will enhance your focus and concentration, allowing you to perform better in your academic endeavors.

Seeking Support:

Dental studies can be mentally and emotionally challenging, and it is essential to seek support when needed. Reach out to your professors, classmates, and mentors for guidance and advice. Join study groups to collaborate and share knowledge. Additionally, consider joining dental associations and attending conferences to network with professionals in your field. Surrounding yourself with a supportive community will help you navigate the challenges and stay motivated throughout your academic journey.

Setting Realistic Goals:

Setting realistic goals is crucial for achieving academic success. Break down your long-term goals into smaller, manageable tasks. Celebrate each milestone you achieve, as this will boost your motivation and confidence. Remember that success is a gradual process, and setbacks are a natural part of the journey. Embrace challenges as opportunities for growth and keep pushing forward.

Conclusion:

By implementing effective time management strategies, maintaining a healthy lifestyle, seeking support, and setting realistic goals, you can overcome dental challenges and achieve academic success. Remember to stay focused, stay motivated, and never lose sight of your passion for dentistry. With determination and perseverance, you have the potential to become a successful dental professional.

# Chapter 7: Exploring Future Trends in Cosmetic Dentistry for Students

## Advancements in Teeth Whitening Technology

In recent years, the field of dentistry has witnessed remarkable advancements in teeth whitening technology, revolutionizing the way we enhance and restore the aesthetics of our smiles. As students aspiring to enter the world of dentistry, it is crucial to stay informed about the latest breakthroughs in this field. This subchapter will delve into the exciting advancements that have emerged in teeth whitening technology, providing you with a comprehensive understanding of the tools and techniques used in modern cosmetic dentistry.

One of the most significant advancements in teeth whitening technology is the development of laser teeth whitening. This procedure utilizes a high-intensity laser to activate a whitening gel applied to the teeth, resulting in a faster and more effective whitening process. Laser teeth whitening offers several advantages, including reduced treatment time, enhanced precision, and longer-lasting results compared to traditional methods.

Another noteworthy advancement is the introduction of LED teeth whitening systems. These systems employ light-emitting diodes (LEDs) to accelerate the whitening process. LED teeth whitening is not only safe and efficient but also more comfortable for patients, as it minimizes sensitivity and gum irritation commonly experienced with other techniques. This advancement has made teeth whitening more accessible and convenient for individuals seeking a brighter smile.

Furthermore, the development of at-home teeth whitening kits has transformed the way people approach teeth whitening. These kits typically include customized trays and professional-grade whitening gel, allowing individuals to whiten their teeth in the comfort of their own homes. At-home teeth whitening kits provide a cost-effective alternative to in-office treatments, making teeth whitening more affordable and accessible to a broader range of patients.

Additionally, advancements in teeth whitening technology have led to the formulation of more advanced whitening agents. These new whitening gels contain ingredients that not only remove surface stains but also penetrate the tooth enamel to target deep-set discoloration. This ensures more comprehensive and long-lasting results, giving patients a brighter and more radiant smile.

In conclusion, the advancements in teeth whitening technology have revolutionized the field of cosmetic dentistry, providing more efficient, comfortable, and accessible options for patients seeking a brighter smile. As students in the field of dentistry, it is crucial to stay up-to-date with these advancements, as they will form the foundation of your future practice. By embracing these innovative techniques and technologies, you will be equipped to offer your patients the most effective and cutting-edge teeth whitening solutions available.

# Innovative Techniques in Dental Veneers and Implants

As students pursuing a career in dentistry, it is crucial to stay updated with the latest advancements in cosmetic procedures. One area that has seen remarkable progress is the field of dental veneers and implants. These innovative techniques have revolutionized the way dentists restore smiles and improve oral health. In this subchapter, we will delve into the exciting world of dental veneers and implants, exploring the cutting-edge techniques that are shaping the future of dentistry.

Dental veneers are thin shells made of porcelain or composite resin that are bonded to the front surface of teeth. They provide a natural-looking solution for correcting a range of dental imperfections, such as chipped, stained, or misaligned teeth. Traditional veneers require the removal of a significant amount of tooth enamel, but thanks to advancements in technology, minimally invasive veneers are now available. These ultra-thin veneers require little to no tooth preparation, preserving the natural structure of the teeth while delivering exceptional aesthetics.

Another area where innovation is thriving is dental implants. Implants are titanium screws that are surgically placed into the jawbone to serve as artificial tooth roots. They provide a permanent solution for replacing missing teeth, offering stability, functionality, and a natural appearance. Over the years, implant technology has advanced significantly, with the introduction of materials like zirconia, which is both durable and aesthetically pleasing. Additionally, computer-aided design and manufacturing (CAD/CAM) technology has revolutionized the implant process, allowing for precise planning and placement, reducing surgery time, and enhancing patient outcomes.

One of the most exciting advancements in dental implants is the concept of immediate loading or same-day implants. Traditionally, implants required a healing period of several months before the final restoration could be placed. However, with immediate loading, a temporary crown or bridge can be attached to the implant on the same day of surgery, significantly reducing treatment time and improving patient satisfaction.

As students, it is important to understand these innovative techniques in dental veneers and implants, as they represent the future of cosmetic dentistry. By staying informed about the latest advancements, we can provide our future patients with the highest level of care and offer them the most effective and efficient solutions for their dental needs. Embracing these techniques will not only enhance our skills as dentists but also contribute to the brighter side of dentistry by transforming smiles and improving the quality of life for our patients.

# The Role of Cosmetic Dentistry in Students' Career Success

In today's competitive world, where appearances matter more than ever, students need to invest in every aspect of their personal branding. One often overlooked aspect is their oral health and the role it plays in their overall appearance. Cosmetic dentistry, a branch of dentistry focused on improving the aesthetics of smiles, can have a significant impact on students' career success.

First impressions are crucial, especially in job interviews or networking events. When meeting someone new, the first thing they notice is your smile. A bright, confident smile can create a positive and lasting impression, making you more memorable to potential employers, professors, or colleagues. By investing in cosmetic dentistry procedures like teeth whitening, veneers, or orthodontics, students can enhance their smiles, boost their self-confidence, and leave a remarkable impression.

Moreover, a healthy and attractive smile can improve students' overall self-esteem. Feeling good about oneself and exuding confidence are essential qualities that can help students excel in their studies and professional endeavors. With increased self-assurance, students are more likely to actively participate in class discussions, engage with professors, and take on leadership roles in extracurricular activities. These experiences can significantly contribute to their personal growth and set them apart from their peers.

Cosmetic dentistry can also address dental issues that may hinder students' career prospects. Misaligned teeth or bite problems can cause difficulties in speech or pronunciation, undermining effective communication skills. By seeking orthodontic treatments or Invisalign, students can correct these issues, improving their speech clarity and articulation, which are critical for presentations, public speaking, and effective communication in any professional setting.

Furthermore, cosmetic dentistry can help students overcome dental insecurities that might hinder their professional growth. Many students struggle with dental flaws such as stained or chipped teeth, gaps, or uneven smiles. These imperfections can affect their self-esteem and make them hesitant to engage in social or professional situations. Cosmetic dentistry procedures like dental bonding, porcelain veneers, or dental implants can effectively address these concerns, providing students with a smile they can proudly showcase, boosting their confidence and allowing them to fully embrace their potential.

In conclusion, cosmetic dentistry plays a vital role in students' career success by enhancing their smiles, boosting self-confidence, improving communication skills, and addressing dental insecurities. Investing in one's oral health not only leads to a more aesthetically pleasing smile but also improves overall well-being and opens doors to greater opportunities. So, students, take charge of your future by embracing the power of cosmetic dentistry and unlock the brighter side of your dental journey!

# Chapter 8: Empowering Students with a Beautiful Smile

## Building Confidence and Self-esteem through Cosmetic Dentistry

Introduction:

In today's society, appearance plays a significant role in how individuals perceive themselves and how they are perceived by others. As students pursuing a career in dentistry, it is crucial to recognize the impact that a confident smile can have on an individual's self-esteem and overall well-being. Cosmetic dentistry offers a range of procedures that can enhance the appearance of teeth and contribute to building confidence. In this subchapter, we will explore the various ways in which cosmetic dentistry can empower students to improve their own self-esteem and help their future patients achieve a brighter smile.

Boosting Confidence:

A confident smile can have a transformative effect on a person's self-confidence. As students in the field of dentistry, we have the unique opportunity to not only improve our own self-esteem but also provide this life-changing experience to our patients. By learning about and practicing cosmetic dentistry, we can gain the skills to address aesthetic concerns such as stained, misaligned, or missing teeth, helping individuals regain their confidence and improve their quality of life.

Enhancing Self-esteem:

Cosmetic dentistry offers a range of procedures that can address various dental concerns. Teeth whitening, for example, is a popular procedure that can brighten a smile and remove stains caused by lifestyle choices or aging. By offering this service to our patients, we can help them feel more confident in their appearance, leading to improved self-esteem and a positive self-image.

Addressing Dental Imperfections:

Crooked or misaligned teeth can be a source of embarrassment for many individuals. As dental professionals, we can learn about orthodontic treatments such as braces and clear aligners, which can straighten teeth and correct bite issues. By providing these services, we can help our patients achieve a beautiful smile, eliminating any self-consciousness they may have had about their dental imperfections.

Replacing Missing Teeth:

Missing teeth can significantly impact a person's self-esteem and ability to function properly. Learning about dental implants and other tooth replacement options allows us to provide our patients with a solution that restores their smile and confidence. By mastering these procedures, we can help individuals regain their ability to chew, speak, and smile without hesitation.

Conclusion:

As students in the field of dentistry, understanding the transformative impact of cosmetic dentistry on self-esteem is essential. By familiarizing ourselves with the various procedures available, we can help our future patients overcome dental imperfections, boost their confidence, and improve their overall quality of life. By building our own self-esteem through cosmetic dentistry, we can better empathize with our patients, providing them with the care and attention they need to achieve their own brighter smiles.

## The Psychological Impact of a Bright Smile on Academic Performance

In today's highly competitive academic environment, students are constantly seeking ways to gain an edge and improve their performance. While traditional methods like studying harder and managing time efficiently are crucial, there is one often overlooked factor that can significantly impact academic success – a bright smile. Yes, you read that right! The condition of your teeth and the confidence it brings can have a profound psychological impact on your overall well-being and academic performance.

Research has shown that a confident smile can boost self-esteem, increase motivation, and enhance cognitive abilities. When you are happy with your smile, you are more likely to feel confident when interacting with peers and professors. This confidence can translate into better classroom participation and increased engagement, leading to improved academic performance.

A bright smile also has the power to positively influence how others perceive you. People with attractive smiles are often perceived as more intelligent, trustworthy, and competent, which can have a significant impact on your academic and professional relationships. When you feel good about your smile, you exude confidence, and others are more likely to take notice and treat you with respect.

Furthermore, maintaining good oral hygiene, including regular visits to the dentist, can also have a positive impact on your overall health. Poor oral health has been linked to various physical and mental health conditions, including cardiovascular diseases and depression. By taking care of your teeth, you are not only improving your smile but also safeguarding your overall well-being, which is essential for academic success.

To achieve a bright smile, it is crucial to prioritize dental care and consider cosmetic dentistry procedures if necessary. From teeth whitening to orthodontic treatments, there are a plethora of options available to help you achieve that confident smile you desire. Consulting with a dentist specializing in cosmetic procedures will allow you to explore the best options tailored to your specific needs and budget.

In conclusion, the psychological impact of a bright smile on academic performance should not be underestimated. By investing in your dental health and ensuring you have a confident smile, you are fostering positive self-perception, boosting self-esteem, and enhancing your overall academic potential. Remember, a bright smile is not just about aesthetics, but a gateway to a brighter academic future!

**Spreading Smiles: Encouraging Others to Embrace Cosmetic Dentistry**

Introduction:

In recent years, cosmetic dentistry has gained significant popularity. More and more people are realizing the importance of a beautiful smile and the positive impact it can have on their self-esteem and overall well-being. As students pursuing a career in dentistry, it is crucial for us to understand the significance of cosmetic dentistry and encourage others to embrace its benefits.

Understanding Cosmetic Dentistry:

Cosmetic dentistry involves a wide range of procedures aimed at improving the aesthetics of a person's smile. From teeth whitening to veneers, dental implants to orthodontics, these procedures can transform a person's smile, enhancing their confidence and quality of life.

Importance of a Beautiful Smile:

A bright and confident smile can open doors to endless opportunities. It can boost self-esteem, improve personal relationships, and even enhance professional success. As future dentists, we need to emphasize the importance of a beautiful smile to our patients and educate them on the various cosmetic dentistry options available.

Breaking the Stigma:

Cosmetic dentistry has often been associated with vanity or unnecessary indulgence. However, it is crucial to break this stigma and educate others about the broader benefits of these procedures. By spreading awareness about the positive impact cosmetic dentistry can have on both physical and mental health, we can encourage more individuals to consider these treatments.

Enhancing Patients' Quality of Life:

Many people suffer from dental issues that affect their quality of life. Crooked teeth, stained enamel, or missing teeth can cause embarrassment and hinder social interactions. By embracing cosmetic dentistry, individuals can regain their confidence and improve their overall well-being. As future dentists, we have the power to transform lives and help our patients achieve a healthy, beautiful smile.

Promoting Preventive Care:

While cosmetic dentistry focuses on enhancing the aesthetics of a smile, it is vital to emphasize the importance of preventive care. Educating our patients on maintaining good oral hygiene, regular dental visits, and preventive measures can help them avoid severe dental issues in the future. By combining preventive care with cosmetic dentistry, we can ensure long-lasting, healthy smiles for our patients.

Conclusion:

As students in the field of dentistry, it is our responsibility to spread awareness and encourage others to embrace the benefits of cosmetic dentistry. By understanding the importance of a beautiful smile and the positive impact it can have on an individual's life, we can educate our patients and help them achieve the smile they desire. Let us embrace cosmetic dentistry as a means to enhance both physical and mental well-being and pave the way for brighter, more confident smiles.

# Chapter 9: Conclusion

## Recap of Key Learnings for Students

As students pursuing a career in dentistry, it is vital to constantly update our knowledge and stay aware of the latest advancements and techniques in the field. In this subchapter, we will recapitulate the key learnings from our journey through "The Brighter Side of Dentistry: Cosmetic Procedures for Students" to ensure that we have a solid foundation in cosmetic dentistry.

Firstly, we have learned about the significance of dental aesthetics and how it can positively impact a patient's self-confidence and overall well-being. Understanding the importance of a beautiful smile and its impact on a person's life is crucial for any aspiring dentist.

We have delved into the various cosmetic procedures available in dentistry, such as teeth whitening, veneers, dental implants, and orthodontics. Each procedure has its unique benefits and considerations, and it is important to evaluate them based on the patient's individual needs and desires.

Furthermore, we have explored the diagnostic techniques used in cosmetic dentistry, including smile analysis, digital imaging, and mock-ups. These tools allow us to visualize the desired outcome and effectively communicate with our patients, ensuring their satisfaction with the final results.

One of the key takeaways from this book has been the emphasis on ethical considerations in cosmetic dentistry.

We have learned the importance of informed consent, patient autonomy, and the need for realistic expectations. It is crucial to prioritize the patient's well-being over financial gain and always provide honest recommendations.

Additionally, we have gained an understanding of the importance of continuous learning and staying updated with the latest advancements in cosmetic dentistry. Technology is constantly evolving, and it is our responsibility to embrace these changes to provide the best possible care to our patients.

Lastly, we have explored the significance of building strong relationships with our patients. Effective communication, empathy, and trust are essential in establishing a successful dental practice. The book has highlighted the importance of creating a comfortable and welcoming environment for our patients, ensuring their satisfaction and loyalty.

In conclusion, "The Brighter Side of Dentistry: Cosmetic Procedures for Students" has provided us with valuable insights into cosmetic dentistry. By recapping the key learnings from this book, we have reinforced our knowledge and equipped ourselves to excel in the field of dentistry. Remember, the pursuit of excellence is a lifelong journey, and by continuously expanding our knowledge, we can provide the best possible care for our patients and make a positive impact on their lives.

## Encouragement to Explore Cosmetic Dentistry and its Benefits

Introduction:
As students in the field of dentistry, you have embarked on a fascinating journey that offers numerous opportunities to improve people's oral health and enhance their smiles. One area of dentistry that is gaining popularity and recognition is cosmetic dentistry. In this subchapter, we will explore the exciting world of cosmetic dentistry and discuss the benefits it offers not only to patients but also to you as future dental professionals.

Enhancing                                                             Smiles:
Cosmetic dentistry focuses on enhancing the aesthetics of a person's smile. Through various procedures, such as teeth whitening, veneers, dental bonding, and orthodontics, cosmetic dentists can transform a person's smile, boosting their self-confidence and improving their overall quality of life. By learning about and offering these procedures, you will have the power to positively impact your patients' self-esteem and contribute to their happiness.

Modern             Techniques           and             Technology:
Advancements in dental technology have revolutionized the field of cosmetic dentistry. From digital smile design to computer-aided manufacturing of dental restorations, these modern techniques allow for precise and predictable results. By embracing these tools, you will not only stay up-to-date with the latest advancements but also have the opportunity to work with cutting-edge technology that makes your work more efficient and effective.

Career                                          Advancement:
By exploring cosmetic dentistry, you open doors to a rewarding career path. Specializing in this field can set you apart from other dental professionals and provide you with a competitive edge in the job market. Additionally, as cosmetic dentistry becomes more popular, the demand for skilled professionals in this niche continues to increase. By adding cosmetic dentistry skills to your repertoire, you can expand your practice and attract a wider range of patients.

Educational                                 Opportunities:
Learning about cosmetic dentistry will broaden your knowledge and skill set. This field requires a deep understanding of dental anatomy, materials, and techniques. By delving into cosmetic dentistry, you will gain knowledge that can benefit your patients in various dental procedures, even those unrelated to aesthetics. Furthermore, attending workshops, conferences, and continuing education courses will allow you to stay updated with the latest trends and techniques in the field.

Conclusion:
As students in the field of dentistry, exploring cosmetic dentistry can be an exciting and rewarding endeavor. By enhancing your patients' smiles, utilizing modern techniques and technology, advancing your career, and expanding your knowledge, you will be well-equipped to make a significant impact on your patients' lives. Embrace the world of cosmetic dentistry, and unlock a world of possibilities for both your patients and yourself.

## Inspiring Students to Embrace the Brighter Side of Dentistry

Dentistry is an incredible field that offers a multitude of opportunities for students to make a positive impact on people's lives. From restoring smiles to improving oral health, dentistry plays a crucial role in enhancing overall well-being. However, many students may have preconceived notions about dentistry that prevent them from fully embracing its brighter side. This subchapter aims to inspire students to look beyond these misconceptions and discover the true beauty and rewards that dentistry has to offer.

One common misconception is that dentistry is solely about drilling and filling cavities. While this is an essential part of dental care, modern dentistry has evolved to encompass a range of cosmetic procedures that can transform patients' lives. From teeth whitening to veneers and orthodontics, dentistry now offers students the opportunity to create stunning smiles and boost patients' self-esteem. By understanding the power of a confident smile, students can unlock the potential of dentistry to positively impact their patients' lives.

Moreover, dentistry is not just about treating ailments; it is about prevention and education. As future dental professionals, students have the chance to educate patients on proper oral hygiene practices, dietary choices, and lifestyle habits that can prevent dental issues. By promoting preventive care, students can empower patients to take control of their oral health and avoid costly and painful procedures in the future.

Furthermore, dentistry is a field that constantly evolves and embraces new technologies and innovations. Students who choose dentistry as their career path will have the opportunity to stay at the forefront of these advancements. From digital dentistry to laser treatments, the field is continuously evolving, providing students with a chance to be part of groundbreaking techniques that improve patient outcomes and make dental procedures more comfortable and efficient.

Finally, dentistry offers a unique blend of art and science. Students can tap into their creative side by designing custom smiles, creating natural-looking restorations, and crafting dentures that perfectly match their patients' facial features. The ability to combine technical skills with artistic talent sets dentistry apart from other healthcare professions and allows students to express their creativity while improving patients' lives.

In conclusion, dentistry is a field brimming with opportunities for students to make a positive impact and embrace the brighter side of oral health care. By dispelling misconceptions, students can unlock the true potential of dentistry to transform smiles, educate patients on preventive care, embrace cutting-edge technologies, and tap into their artistic abilities. Dentistry offers a fulfilling and rewarding career that allows students to leave a lasting impression on their patients' lives. Embrace the brighter side of dentistry and embark on a journey that will not only enhance your professional growth but also bring smiles to countless faces.